Family Conflict

By: Lisa Bedrick

Dedication:

I dedicate this book to my sweetie. I love you so much Zach! Thank you for providing a perfect and peaceful life for me finally. You have been such a great friend and lover. I have never felt closer to someone than how I feel with you. You are awesome!

Conflict

The cause of pretty much every conflict, and most parting of the ways of two people, is when two people want two totally different things.

For example, and this is a sad analogy, but my dad wanted to get physical with me as a kid, but I didn't obviously. So that created conflict and a parting of the ways for us.

My ex wanted me to have a 3rd kid, because he was dying to have a son. I didn't really want to. That was probably the main reason we parted ways. I figured the two lovely girls I already gave him should have been enough.

My ex mother in law really wanted to vaccinate my girls. I didn't want that, at all. So we stopped being friends because of that.

The only thing my best friend and I have conflicted over is I think she should try online dating, but she really doesn't want to. Otherwise we agree on pretty much anything. That is why we have stayed friends for 23 years.

My mom and I haven't conflicted on too much. I didn't really want her to marry my step dad but she did anyways. Once she was married, I didn't disagree with her over it anymore. It was already done.

Anytime two people want two very different things, there will be conflict. The way to avoid this is to pretty much never want anything, at least not a lot.

Watch out for wanting something that is totally different from what others want, within reason. If you know what is best, stick with that. Maybe you can change the mind of the other person to want what you want. If you can't, just let it go. Whatever you want so bad, just let it go. Then you will never have conflict ever again. Very nice.

Women Have Lost

I wrote a book about Feminism called Feminism Sucks. I was analyzing how most women have to decide between a career or raising kids. The issue in our modern world though is that women are doing both. So many women have abandoned the home and instead focus on making money. Then others don't respect them, and they don't respect themselves as much. It is like they are running away. They don't want to clean their house. They want to pay someone else to clean it. They don't want to raise their kids. They want a nanny or a daycare to raise their kids. No daycare worker will care about your kids as much as you do.

Women are leaving their natural duties to chase money. What do they have in the end? They feel less in touch with their kids. Kids are now running wild because too many women are chasing money instead of bonding with their kids.

Whatever you want to buy, is it really that important? Aren't your kids more important?

We wonder why kids are so messed up these days. It is because their mothers have run away from them. They are home but not really home. Or they are just never home.

Stay home women. Raise your kids yourself. No amount of money can replace the time with your kids. Before you know it, they will be gone. You will wish you would have focused on them more and not money.

Men, step it up and provide well for your families. If you want your wife to do a great job raising the kids, then you have to do a great job providing for them. You can do it. I believe in you.

Family Stealing

About 2 months ago my boyfriend's grandma was stolen from. I think it was her daughter that did it. The daughter stole 16k out of her home safe. Why does she even have a home safe? Both him and his mom said she has it because she doesn't trust banks. Now she knows she can't trust her daughter. I wanted to say something, but what can you say when things like that happen? I chose to just watch the bonfire from a big distance so I wouldn't get burned too.

She was accusing everyone of stealing it, except me. The entire thing may have been in her head because she is 83 years old, but I think it really happened. Her daughter hasn't worked in quite awhile, and she had no savings. Her ex husband stole all of her savings. Her mom was providing for her, but maybe she felt like it was not enough, so she stole. Also she will get half of the inheritance from her mom so she may have felt that was her money anyway. It was still wrong though. I hope she realizes that. I don't get why they are still friends after that. I would not be able to forgive that, but I guess we can forgive anything if we want to.

I told my boyfriend after the incident that if this is a recurring thing, it is like women who are beat by their man. They should leave but they love their man too much and stay. Everyone around wonders why, but it must be that they are stupid. It is hard to respect people who let that happen to them. Then they have few friends because everyone is frustrated by them allowing that. This situation was like that. I was frustrated she allowed that, and didn't confront her daughter.

If someone hurts you or steals from you etc, I hope you respect yourself enough to distance yourself from them. You do not deserve to be treated badly. You treat people how to treat you. What you allow is what will happen. Don't let others hurt you, and get away with it. Put some distance there so it won't happen again.

Jealousy Over Children

I think it is very common that husbands are jealous of the love between a mother and a son. Women also get jealous of the love between a father and a daughter.

Perhaps each parent wonders if that kid will replace them emotionally someday. That happens quite often. A woman might love her son more than her man. A father may begin to love his daughter more than his wife.

Obviously that is not good if that happens. I heard in sermons a lot, "A marriage is forever. Kids are only for 18 years. You need to love your spouse more than you love your kids." Also if you forget about loving your spouse and focus on the kids, that marriage won't last very long.

It is always a balancing act for every mom. She needs to try showing equal love to her man and her kids. It can be quite tricky to do that.

I named my son James. I realized after that the meaning of that name is "supplanter" or replacer. To me that means it could be easy for me to let my baby boy replace my man in my heart. I need to watch out for that.

Spouses are supposed to be the first priority, then children.

The love a parent has for their child needs to be in light of knowing they won't be around forever. Someday they will fall in love and run away from you, emotionally. That transition will be a lot smoother if you don't let them into your heart too much in the first place. Then you will be more ok with them falling in love and leaving you.

When it is time to, let your kids go. Realize that your call to parent is only temporary. Always and forever keep your mate as your first priority. They deserve that.

Motherhood

 I have always enjoyed watching cat moms be moms. My first experience with it was when I was about 9 years old. My cat Tiger had three perfect kittens. Two white ones and an orange striped one like her. Then a year later she had another litter of 5 kittens. I had a cat in my former house who had 3 litters. They were all adorable. I sold most of the kittens on Craigslist for like $20 each.

There is nothing cuter than getting to watch kittens grow up. They wrestle and climb trees and purr a lot when you hold them

I think this mommy cat is having a hard time being a mom. But I'm sure it's hard to lay 24/7 with your babies and let them nurse on you. That is a big reason I did mainly formula with my two daughters. I didn't want to feel stuck in bed nursing all day. If my cat Princess could talk, I think she would tell me, "I want to be free and to run around." I would say back to her, "Nope you stay with your kittens." In my last litter of kittens, the mom cat would sometimes leave the backyard and I would worry if she would come back. When I would call out for her she would come back. One time I scolded her and said, "I give you milk and chicken. Why can't you just stay back here?"

With this mom cat, I had her since she was a baby a year ago. We have a pretty good friendship. Hopefully we will enjoy being co-parents of these kittens.

Why Divorce Happens

 Half of all marriages end in divorce. Why is that? I think it's because men don't understand women and women don't understand men. Women don't understand why men love to drink and smoke in excess. Men don't understand why women love to spend tons of money. Women don't understand why men are always thinking about sex. Men don't understand why women almost never think about sex. It's because we have to deal with the pain. Men just get to enjoy the fun part of procreating.

Women don't understand why men are so attached to their mom or grandma. Men don't understand why women aren't super close to their family. It's because we like being independent and grown up.

Both genders don't understand why the other gets fat really easily. We don't get why we all can't look like movie stars forever. We can't because movie stars barely eat anything. I don't know how they do it.

They have millions of dollars but are barely allowed to eat anything. That must get super frustrating for them.

Women don't understand why men obsess over their cars or trucks. Men don't understand why women keep buying more home decoration things. It's because we have to look at our house 24/7 and we like it to look very nice and happy.

Women don't understand why some men watch porn for hours. Men don't understand why women can do online shopping for hours. Both are just something to do so we aren't bored. Both can be destructive to a marriage, but most people think their marriage will never end, so they do stupid things like that.

If both genders would try to understand each other better, there would be less divorces. Maybe in the future we can all try to understand each other more.

Getting Help from Parents

 Why do children with rich parents end up doing drugs? Why are they usually less responsible with money? Maybe it's because they feel they can never fill the shoes of their parents, so they give up before they even try.

I have noticed that weak parents produce strong children. Strong parents tend to produce weak children. Why is that? When there are strong parents, or rich parents, the kids think the parent will always catch them when they fall, so they feel totally ok with falling a lot. When the parents are weak the child is more cautious about falling, because they don't know if anyone will catch them.

I have been in both situations. I had a single mom for 7 years. Then she married my step-dad and I had rich parents, at least kind of rich. I probably became more careless with money because I always felt they could give me money if I needed it. They were my safety net. I used to always say, "My mom is my savings account." But lately she has been weak. She hasn't worked in about 10 years, but she deserved to retire early due to having scoliosis. My step-dad has money, but he isn't really my dad, so I don't feel entitled to it in any way.

Since my mom has not been working, I have become stronger. I have been fending for myself. I have tried hard to keep myself from needing their help. When I separated from my ex, I needed help for a few months but then I figured out how to care for myself. I had to give up my kids so I could stop being dependent on my parents. I probably could have gotten government assistance, but I don't really like doing that.

It is tricky when you need help from your parents. Ideally none of us ever should. Emergencies happen but then we need to get back up and run for ourselves again.

Submit to One Another

Before Paul said wives are meant to submit to their husbands, he said "submit to one another." Men were also told to submit to their woman. Most men have a hard time doing this.

Paul also said, "Those who marry will face many troubles in this life." The trouble comes when there is no submission on both sides. Either the wife or the husband remains stubborn. They refuse to do what their mate wants them to do. Then a power struggle might start. People often react in anger or isolation when they don't get their way. They either use anger to control the other person, or they pout and withhold love when they don't get what they want.

The solution is to do almost everything your mate wants you to do. If you don't, your relationship, and your life, will be more stressful.

As kids, many of us rebelled against our parents. As adults, a lot of us rebel against our mate. Don't do that. It can be fun, in a way, but also it is stressful. The forbidden fruit seems sweeter until you make your mate mad.

Learn to fall in line. Do what your mate wants you to do, within reason, and your life will go a lot better.

Respect Yourself

 So many people put up with so much abuse. They either abuse themselves or let others abuse them. I remember reading that sexual abuse victims feel like damaged goods. It is common for abuse victims to let one person after another hurt them, because their self-esteem is low.

If you don't really like yourself, you will let all kinds of bad things happen to you. You will over eat and hurt yourself that way. You will allow verbal abuse toward you to occur often.

I had a co-worker who kept letting her boyfriend hit her. Every day almost he would beat her up a lot. To be fair she beat him up too. I didn't get why she kept letting that happen. I figured maybe it was their entertainment instead of watching movies. I think it mainly was due to low self-respect. They both did some kind of drugs too, so that was another way they disrespected themselves.

On the Jay Shetty show yesterday I heard a great quote. "Don't let grief be an excuse to hurt yourself." It made me think how I started smoking cigarettes after I lost my daughters. I did not smoke when I was pregnant though. Praise God for helping me to respect myself and my baby then.

When we miss someone we might hurt ourselves. We blame ourselves for them being gone so we lose respect for ourselves and hurt ourselves. Don't do that.

Forgive yourself. Whatever you need to forgive yourself for, forgive it. Not every choice in life is easy. Most things are out of your control. We can't do much about what others decided to do or what they wanted. You have to just let things go sometimes. You have to let people go sometimes. Most things will not last forever. You can hope that they will, but realistically life is very unpredictable. Always be ready for anything. Then you won't have a mid-life crisis when things go bad. You will be mentally ready for it.

There is a fine line though between expecting bad things and realizing that they might happen. If you expect bad, you might cause it. If you realize bad things might happen, you have a back-up plan. You are prepared for anything.

Respect yourself. No matter what you have done, you deserve to be treated well simply because you are a human. And let the past go.

Focus on the Family

One reason I write books and put out so much info to the world is that Focus on the Family saved me. My mom grew stronger through listening to them on the radio. When my dad attempted to rape me at age 6 she called them to get prayer. They reported it, and that spared me from things being ongoing with my dad. He went to jail and never was able to abuse me ever again. Praise God.

Thank God for Focus on the Family. They still have great videos on YouTube that will help anyone. Look them up and watch some.

If you know any child or person being abused, give them a place to live. Help them to escape and get safe.

May God heal you all from any abuse that you endured.

A Pay Back

 I used to tell my ex that when my girls grew up and got married we could live with them. I said that could be our retirement. He said that was stupid. I was thinking after all the waking up in the middle of the night for them, that didn't seem stupid to me.

All kids do owe their parents. They kept you alive for 18 years and provided all your needs. That is why God said, "Honor your mother and father."

I used to struggle with that given my dad and step-dad were child predators. It is never totally easy to honor your parents, but it's good in the long run if you can.

If your parent needs anything, you should help them, if you are able to do so.

The issue in our modern world is most parents are so rich, their kids know they won't have to help them. I suppose that is both a blessing and sad. Then families stay far apart when no one needs anyone else.

This is why poor families are somewhat cute. They all help each other a lot, because they all need help at some point. My grandma had to help my mom a lot when she was a single mom. I'm sure she appreciated her daughter asking for help. But now we all are so independent. Most people don't need other people for anything. This causes an isolation that causes the depression issue in our society. Very sad.

Over Eating

A lot of people stress eat when they have conflict. My uncle told me a while ago, people eat in place of love or in defense of love. His wife was always over weight, but he stayed with her anyways and still loved her. I always loved that about him.

To eat in place of love is to eat your feelings. You are stressed out so you use food like a drug to feel better. You need a hug, but you eat a cookie instead.

To eat in defense of love is to get fat to ensure no one will love you. Maybe you feel uncomfortable being loved. Maybe you hate the opposite sex staring at you. You want your mate to reject you, so you get fat to ensure they will. Maybe physical contact is awkward for you. Maybe your mate pursues you too much. You want them to want you less, so you get fat.

A friend in college said she always wondered why the fall of man happened via eating. What did that show? Eating can lead us into great sin perhaps?

I always have had a hard time respecting pastors who are very large. My thinking has been, if they have no self control with food, then do they have any self control? If they have no self control, how can anyone say they are actually Christian?

A basic sign a person is a Christian is their ability to have self control. You can say no to sin. It is possible. The Holy Spirit gives any believer the ability to have self control and to sin less. If you cannot say no to sin, even the sin of over eating, you can't say you have the Holy Spirit in you.

"Test yourself to see if you are in the faith," Paul said.

I hope you all will try to have more self control in all areas of your life. You can do it. Just believe you can and then you can.

Unplanned Parenthood

Here are my thoughts on the importance of pregnancy prevention.

So many people criticize Planned Parenthood, but I would say they do a good job helping poor moms not have to many kids. I recommend birth control pills over abortions, of course. The pull out method is the best way to prevent pregnancy. Of course, what every woman needs to do is set boundaries with whatever man she is sleeping with. She needs to tell him that he has to pull out, unless he won the lottery lately. But too often women don't say what they need. They want to have fun, but maybe they can't provide for a child. Ideally anyone who can't afford a child should not be having sex, but for those who do, the woman needs to make it clear she wants the man to pull out.

I was just watching Aladdin again, and that got me thinking about this problem in our world. There are starving children at the beginning of the movie. It made me think, "Why does that happen? Why are there starving children?" It happens when the father isn't willing to work hard enough, or the woman is not willing to leave the man if he won't work hard enough.

Men, you need to provide well for any amount of sperm you decide to shoot out. If you don't want to work hard, then don't ever have sex. Wouldn't that be great if that was a rule all men had to follow?

I have known a few men who didn't want to work hard enough to provide for their kids. They should have never had sex in the first place. You can't have the fun without putting in the hard work. Well you can, but you should not be allowed to.

If men, and women, can't afford children, they should abstain from sex entirely.

Over the Limit

 My boyfriend has a drinking problem. That is why I haven't married him yet, and he is still my boyfriend.

Is it ever wise to drink? Probably not. Can it be beneficial? It might be.

I used to drink a Truly drink every night after work. I worked at Papa John's and it was very stressful. I felt I needed the drink to calm my anxiety down so I could sleep. It also replaced me having dinner, which was nice, since I don't like to cook. I mainly eat pre-made salads for my meals.

If you drink, what is your reason? Do you ever feel guilty about drinking?

In the New Testament there is only one command regarding drinking. Paul said, "Do not get drunk with wine for that is debauchery." But when are you drunk? You probably know when you are. Why did Paul say this? Because drinking leads to sin, usually. It does not always, but generally it does. That is why Christians really should abstain from alcohol. That is my opinion.

If you wonder if that is best, watch the movie 28 Days with Sandra Bullock. It is great!

Why do men drink in excess? Ok, some women do too. Is it due to stress? Is it because they just want to have fun? Is it actually because they hate their life, and they want to die? Most people don't realize how possible it is to die from drinking too much. Some do it on purpose, others have no idea that death can happen. They are playing with fire. They like to walk on the edge of the cliff and hope they won't fall over the side. This has always been called living on the edge.

People do that with all kinds of things. When they don't value their life, they aren't careful. If you think you have nothing big to live for, why does being careful matter? God said, "Without a vision the people perish." If you don't have a plan or goal for your future, you won't care about living a reckless life.

It also can be just about having fun. For some people, it takes A Lot for them to consider it a fun day. Boredom is horrible to them. It has to be over the top to be fun. That is why some spend excessively with no limit for themselves. Some drink too much. Some eat too much. Others do drugs often.

Try to have a limit for yourself. The older you get, the more you realize the importance of having a limit on how much fun you can have, or how much fun you should have.

In my first marriage I had a problem with buying too many things online. If I wanted it, I got it. All the bills still got paid on time, usually. But I didn't really limit myself very much. Now I have a limit for my spending. All things in moderation, right? It is nice to reward yourself, but not too much. You have to have some fun, or else you will get depressed over not having any fun. But if you have too much fun, you also might feel depressed. You might feel guilty for having too much fun, for going over a limit you should have for yourself.

Find the middle ground. Have some fun but not too much fun. May God give you wisdom on what the middle ground would be for you. God bless.

Hey go buy my book titled Alcoholics and Co-Dependency on Amazon. Search Lisa Bedrick books.

My Big Brother

The grumpiest person I've ever known is my older brother. Maybe it was because he was homeless for a season, a few months. I think he hates women but he was kind of abandoned by his mom and sister, me. He was left to fend for himself from the time he was 18.

I tried having an apartment with him for a while, but his dog made that not doable.

He has always been verbally abusive. I don't get why. I think it's because he has been verbally abused by others a lot. Hurt people hurt people right? I try to be patient with him, but I think it's time for a break from his attitude.

Pray for him, that his heart will melt and stop being so hard. I hope he finds happiness in the rest of his life.

Killers of Love

There has always been someone trying to mess up any relationship I was in.

With my first serious bf Roger it was my mom. I don't know what she said. All I know is she talked to Roger on the phone one day and he said she was really throwing me under the bus. I was like that's great...

Then with my ex-husband my mom said after we face timed her that he seemed a bit stupid but whatever. I stayed with him anyways.

With my next bf, my ex-husband lied and told him I was heavily into drugs after he and I broke up. He told me about it. I was like, "What...only if cigarettes count as drugs. What a jerk. I can't believe he said that to you."

With the next bf my brother said to him that he should not be with me. How rude.

With the next one, my manager told me he looked like a bad boy, and that I needed to get online and find a new man. I just ignored her, for the most part. That probably did cause me to break up with him a few times though.

With my current man, a friend said since he was on medication, I shouldn't be with him. I ignored that too.

I was just thinking how I have never had a blessing in regards to anyone I was with. Very odd. But why do people expect to get a blessing from someone? Usually people are against your relationship because they are jealous and want to break you up.

Just ignore the haters. If you are happy, then stay happy. If you feel peace about being with whoever you are with, then stay with them. No one is perfect. No one will be approved of by all your friends and family, so don't worry about it. Just enjoy your relationship and stay with them if you really love them.

Conflict with My Mom

A big reason why I waited 4 years to have more kids after giving up my last 2 kids was I didn't know if I want to keep my step-dad from seeing my future kids. I have decided it is best if he doesn't see any more of my children. My mom and I didn't really have to discuss it. I suppose how we did discuss it was we talkedc on the phone a while ago. She said what David did with my oldest daughter was just a game. I ended the phone call after that and didn't call her for a few months. I guess I was just thinking I didn't want to talk about that, and the way she said it seemed strange. Why would she call it a game? Why would she think anything sexual with a kid could be a game, and it would be ok? Maybe she didn't get exactly what the game entailed. I don't necessarily know either, but I feel God told me many times it was not something adults should be doing with kids.

Now that I have my 3rd kid I know I don't want my step-dad around him. I wish I would have known that for my first two kids. So far that seems to be ok with my mom. Hopefully it always will be. I don't really want to argue with her about that.

I don't get why my mom is still with him when he has issues like that. I suppose all women put up with something to be with a man, but that is the worst that it could get. A man who wants to play with kids inappropriately to me would be totally off limits. I suppose she just thinks if he isn't around kids, it doesn't matter, and she isn't a kid. I think overall she doesn't know how messed up his brain is in regards to children. I have no idea why he is that way. I just know that he is. I hope someday the light will come on for her and she will escape having to live with him. Maybe she could live with me. I hope God will provide her with the means to get away if she wants to. May she realize someday that he has serious problems.

Money Matters

The main cause of divorce is money issues.

The music video that I think says more than any other video is this one by Katy Perry. She walks into a theme park called Oblivia. The first thing you see is houses hanging by strings. She says, "Yeah we think we're free." As long as you are paying a mortgage, or paying off any debt, you are not free. A Bible verse says, "The borrower is always slave to the lender." But we all choose to not think about that. We rack up credit card debt like it's no big deal, which is a reference to another song of hers. We run on the hamster wheel and think we are getting somewhere, but it is mostly a waste of time. If you buy a house on credit, you pay a ton of interest. If you are paying off any debt, you are mostly paying interest. That is the main message I think she meant to send. She noticed that all her friends who bought homes on credit were hanging by a string with their property. If you can't pay, it's over and you are kicked out. There is no freedom when you owe anyone anything.

I think the rap part says the most,

"Up in your high place, liars

Time is ticking for the empire

The truth they feed is feeble

As so many times before

The greed over the people

They stumbling and fumbling and we about to riot

They woke up, they woke up the lions."

What does this mean? The bankers make tons off of us who are at the bottom. They don't care that we all struggle, run ourselves out on a hamster wheel. They like to see us suffer perhaps. Why would we riot? Interest rates. Most people are oblivious to how much of a rip off any home loan or car loan is. They buy whatever they want and then later regret it. They get buyer's remorse eventually. Is anything we buy really worth it? Things wear out and break down. Is anything worth what we pay for it? Very few things are. I recently bought fake grass which was worth it. :) But the sooner we wake up and see the lie of materialism and consumerism, the happier we will be.

Learn to live with less, because how much do you really need? What you want is way more than what you need.

Don't let yourself become a slave to the system of working and buying and it never stops. Pay off your debts, and then don't get more debt. It's better to drive a 20 year old car then be a slave to a car loan for the next 7 years. Car loans aren't 5 years anymore. They are 7. Watch out. Be careful with the money you spend or commit to. Don't be a hamster running on a wheel forever. Learn to be smarter with the money you spend and save.

Feminism

Here are my thoughts on the music video Flowers by Myley Cyrus. It seems to be about feminism, but it goes beyond that even.

First, she starts out being dressed like mother Mary with the head covering. Then she ties her hair up like all of us modern women do. Then she swims and is working out to tone her body, like most men try to do. If you think about it, working out is mostly a manly thing to do. Then she goes into her ex boyfriend's closet and puts on his clothes. Then she is seen dancing on top of a building like she turned into a crazy man. Maybe it's a reference to King Kong. He was on top of buildings holding defenseless women.

When I first heard the song a year ago, I was like, ok this is good. It's about surviving after a break up. The funny thing is she is the same sign as me and her ex-husband is the same sign as my boyfriend. I bet he was great at taking care of her, like my man is with me. But then they broke up, and of course she missed him. Instead of crying over it, she literally decides to become a man herself. That is the implication in the music video.

She goes from being a sweet docile woman like mother Mary, to turning into King Kong possibly. So her break up made her a warrior rather then made her weaker.

I can say I can relate, my last break up made me a lot stronger too. I went and made my own money and enjoyed my freedom. But that life of being without a man's protection is only good for so long. Eventually all of us women miss the affection and protection of a man, so we are willing to submit to a man again, and that is good. The best life a woman can have is to be with a good man.

Don't believe the lie that you are better without a man. You might be better without a bad man, but not a good man. I'm glad I finally found a good man. Try harder to find a good man, and good luck to you.

Papa John's

Thank God for Papa John's. They helped me get through my hardest time in life. I lost my family due to my ex going insane. I could have ended up like Adam Sandler's character in Reign Over Me except that I had Papa John's.

That place became my new close knit family for 3 years. It was my great love. It was my passion. It brought me tons of joy. I went from having just my bf to having 15 close friends. We laughed and danced and partied, a little. We carried each other's burdens. That place was my gym and my counseling office. It was my food each week and my social life.

I followed my brother's lead in working there. He had worked for a Pizza Hut for about 10 years. I could see why he stuck with it for so long.

I hope someday I'll work at a Papa John's again. It was tons of fun. I even got to be a manager there, which felt so cool. If you need a new and better life, go work at a Papa John's.

God is Love

"God so loved the world that he gave." The more we love, the more we give to others.

Love is not holding a grudge. Love keeps no record of wrongs. Love is patient and kind. It does not envy. It does not boast.

Love is selfless. It is thinking of others above yourself. It is always wanting to serve others and give to others.

It is good to be wise when you give. Don't give so much to the point that you resent what you give. God loves a cheerful giver. If you can't give what you give cheerfully, then don't give at all.

Love benefits others. Love looks out for others. Love protects and provides for others if they are in need. Love does not look out only for his own interest, but also the interests of others.

Love always speaks in a kind manner. Love is calm and gentle.

The more you love something, the more you value it. You take good care of it. If it is your pet, you feed it as much food as it needs. If it is your children, you watch over them well, and feed them as much food as they need.

The opposite of love is selfishness. When you want just what you want, and it doesn't matter what others want. That is not love. That is greed.

Be a loving person. The more loving you are, the more others will respect you and want to be around you, and the better your life will turn out.

Contract Broken

When I first met my bf, I was scared to move forward with him. The last guy I had kids with broke the contract. He was supposed to provide for me forever. That is the usual exchange. A woman gives a man cute kids, and then he promises to provide for her forever. That didn't happen the last time. I can only hope that will happen this time.

When people let you down, it's hard to believe in humanity again. You stop hoping for the best. You stop believing the best is even possible.

If you have experienced lots of disappointments in your life, try to keep your hope alive. Just because one person let you down in a big way, that doesn't mean every person will let you down. There are still a few good people alive today. Find them, and believe that they will be better than those other people.

Cancer

My dad has cancer. This sounds sad, but I was a bit happy when I found out about that. He molested me as a kid. In my opinion, he should have died a long time ago.

I heard once that when a man is caught molesting a child, there could be hundreds of other kids that he molested. He is currently living in an old folks home that his brothers are most likely paying for, because they don't want him to live with them.

I heard a lot on Joyce Meyer videos that she bought a house for her dad when he was old. She was raped by her dad many times. That seemed insane to me. That must have been extremely hard to do. She said God told her to do it. I suppose he did, or she just felt obligated to do it because he didn't have enough money saved for retirement.

I don't think I would do that for my dad, even if I was rich. He is responsible for himself. I am not responsible for him. I might feel like I owe him if he didn't molest me, but he kind of messed up my entire life by doing that, so I do not owe him anything.

If your parents hurt you in a severe way, don't feel like you owe them anything. They need to care for themselves and figure it out. That sounds cold but it's a cold world now. Let them get the karma they deserve.

Heartbreak

 One of my favorite songs when I was young was by Mariah Carey called Heartbreaker. "Heartbreaker you got the best of me, but I just keep on coming back incessantly." It had a fun beat. It made it sound like that was a good idea to do that. No, if someone keeps breaking your heart, you probably should leave them alone, at least for a season. Give them the space they clearly want. The main reason people are mean to other people is because they just want to be left alone for a while. So let them be alone.

I remember one of my exes said to me, "You don't have to start a fight with me just because you need a nap. Just take a nap." That was a good word.

My sister in law has a broken heart now. My brother keeps breaking up with her. He says it's because she doesn't rinse her dishes. That can be pretty annoying when people don't do that, but I'm sure there is more. Over a year ago his dog died. He had that dog for about 14 years since he was a puppy. It was like his second son. He said in that time he felt like he wanted to die. That was the last time he broke up with his lady. I'm sure he just wanted to be alone to grieve.

I was thinking today of the song, "I can't make you love me if you don't. I can't make your heart feel something it won't." That was my song when my ex-husband and I broke up. What the song meant to me was I couldn't make him be nice to me. He was raised to become a jerk because his dad was a jerk. We often are exactly like our parents, no matter how hard we try not to be. My brother is a big time jerk just like our dad was, but I know he doesn't want to be a jerk. He is just following what he saw modeled for his 42 years of life by our dad. My dad really didn't know how to be kind. My brother also has a very hard time knowing how to be kind. They both have been hurt a lot though, so they probably prefer to be alone. They push others away because that is easier to handle. If you are never around other people, no one can hurt you.

If someone is determined to be alone, maybe for their own mental health recovery, they aren't available for love. We all need to heal from something. Sometimes being around others helps us to heal. Other times being alone enables us to heal better and faster. Maybe something you do reminds them of the person they want to forget about. Then they reject you, but really they are rejecting that other person. Like the song by Usher, "You Remind Me." Go listen to it. :)

If someone is rejecting you, just know they probably don't mean to break your heart. They just want to be alone for a while. Sometimes we all just need to be alone.

Nurse Conflict

The very first conflict I had with someone after my baby boy was born was with a nurse. I'm sure she was the reason CPS was set against us. I had a visit from CPS the next morning after dealing with her. They said I was accused of not caring about my baby. I couldn't believe all that happened to me.

The night before I had decided to stay up all night to take care of my baby in the hospital, so I didn't send him to the nursery. I made a pact with myself to stay up off and on until 6am to take care of him to make sure I could do it. I had just had a C Section 3 days before that. I knew when I went home I would have to do the night shift. The night nurse was wary of me keeping my own son all night. She said. "They told me you have high blood pressure." I said, "It's not like I'm just going to pass out." She probably thought I had an attitude with her, so she made up tons of lies about me to tell CPS to cause me trouble. I hope she regrets doing that. And I hope she won't do that to any other moms. Just because she didn't get to be a mom anymore because she was too old, she didn't have to cause issues for a young mother.

I think it was partly a racism thing. She was Mexican and I am white. I am sure she has felt mistreated by some white people simply due to her race, so she wanted to get back at white people in general. Then the CPS lady was Mexican. The case was finally ended when a white CPS lady came to our home to interview the whole family. I figured that was a God send that she was white. Thank God she was able to help us out and close the case.

Racism is so annoying. I am from California. Almost no one is racist there. But here in Texas, there is a lot more racism. It's very sad.

I'm sure you all have stories of racism affecting you. Hopefully you don't, but if you do, may God heal you of the wounds from racism.

My Wonderful Second Chance

About two years ago I hit a deer with my car while on a pizza delivery. It messed up my car so much that it was barely working. The break pedal became almost impossible to push. I asked God why he let that happen to me. He said it was so I would be ready to start a family again. I wasn't ready then, so I sold that car and got a smaller, more fuel efficient car so I could keep doing pizza deliveries. I had to endure a bit more work drama and another demeaning boss before I was ready.

All women have to decide how they will contribute to society. Some do it with having children. Others do it with having a great career that they feel happy doing. I have done almost every job out there. I have seen the world, which I wanted to do before having kids. There is nothing else I wanted to accomplish. So I was ready for family number two to begin.

I resented a few times that I had to start at square one again. My ex refused to work things out with me. He refused to let me see my first two daughters. So I had to start over. I have realized lately though that he and I never really loved each other. He was not capable of love, for whatever reason. I therefore did not love him because I felt he did not love me.

I think as you get older you become more capable of love. When you are young, you don't know what love is. You think love is just passion, but it is generosity and humility. It is forgetting about yourself and putting the other person first. It is never wanting to hurt them in any way. It took me 35 years to figure out love. I suppose some never figure it out.

Family number 2 began in a very difficult way. I had a C Section 2 months ago. It was the hardest week of my life. It all started when my mother in law came over and noticed I looked off. She took my blood pressure and it was very high. She suggested that I go to the hospital. Luckily I was mentally prepared for this. I had been reading about presclampsia and realized that I might have that. My pee had foam in it for awhile, and I realized that probably was not normal. I read that babies can be and should be delivered early in such situations. But I was worried my baby would be in the ICU for awhile. Praise God he came out healthy. He was about 2 weeks early, but he was ok. At first they tried to induce my labor. That wasn't working, so 12 hours after they tried that I had a C section done. I guess before the C Section I said to the nurses, "Can we just get this over with?" So they did. It all seemed like a dream, but it was real. At that point I had been infused with God knows how many drugs. I was not myself. I kept trying to get off my hospital bed before the C Section, but my boyfriend wouldn't let me. He had a very firm look on his face as if to say, "No we are doing this." I'm sure my instincts kicked in and I was thinking, "Why am about to let them cut me open? That is crazy." So I was trying to escape.

But it happened. I had the C Section. The pain was quite annoying afterwards. I had a hard time getting up to pee and walking arond. I was walking like a turtle, which is funny because now I have 5 pet turtles. I wish I could say to them, "I was just like you a little bit ago." I survived though. That is all that matters. They put me on a ton of blood pressure medication that caused me to hallucinate a bit. They were all silly halluciations like worm people falling over each other. I don't recommend that anyone takes that. It really is just acid, I think anyways. Like acid off the street. It did not help my bloood pressure at all. What did help was getting home and sleeping more and eating good foods. God kept telling me to drink lots of juice, so I have been doing that for 2 months now. I just live off of juice, and yogurt and salads. That is how I got my blood pressure back to normal.

I never thought I would have a C Section. Ever since I started my period at 12 I have been horribly afraid of getting pregnant and having a C Section. But I did it. I overcame, and I am very proud of myself for surviving all that. If you ever need a C Section, I promise you too will be ok. Just believe that you will be ok and you will be.

Be a Great Citizen

Here are ways you can serve our great nation...

If you see trash, Pick It Up. Don't worry, it won't give you rabies.

Put your shopping cart back where it should go.

Pick up your dog poop so it won't attract flies.

Be a nice driver.

Hug your family every day. The more hugs, the less angry people we would have running around.

Make pb and j's for homeless people and give them a bottle of water. Maybe that will help them want to work finally so they can then do likewise.

Don't be a litter bug.

Don't let your dogs run around in the street, and keep them quiet.

Never act in a mean way, no matter how pissed off you feel.

If you see stray animals, take them to a shelter.

Keep your grass cut so it looks nice.

Watch only happy things so you can always be happy.

Never yell at anyone. Go take a relaxing bath instead.

I hope you care about America and strive to make it a better place like I do.

My Mom

My entire life I was very scared of my mom's temper. A few times I thought she might kill me. I suppose most kids feel that with their parents. I remember a comedian saying his dad would say, "Boy I brought you into this world and I can take you out."

I never understood why she got so mad. Now I understand it was most likely due to her not eating enough protein. She lived off of sugar. If you do that, your blood sugar is like a roller coaster. You never feel stable. It is easy to feel more emotional. You have to eat meat or cheese more often then you eat carbs and sugar.

I was hesistant to have kids because I didn't know if she would be a good grandma. She was very impatient with me, and I wasn't sure if she would be patient with my kids. She was a bit unstable with my daughters. It was a big disappointment for me. I thought she would be a good grandma, but overall, I would say she was not. She was not very kind to my oldest daughter. I never could figure out why.

She said once that my two daughters reminded her of my brother and I. I should have said, "But they are totally different children." She assumed my oldest girl would end up being slow like my big brother was. I think it's wrong to ever assume something about anyone. You never know what someone will turn out to be like.

It was this negative assumption that started a lot of family drama in my last family. I can only hope there won't be negativity like that in my second attempt at a family.

Don't ever assume you know what your kids will turn out to be like. Let them be innocent until proven guilty. The past doesn't always have to repeat itself unless you assume that it will. Then maybe it will. Hope for the best rather than assume the worst.

Mom Attachment

This may seem odd, but every time my bf talks to his mom in person or texts her I feel jealous. Why do I feel that way? I now know why. Because my ex husband basically left me to go marry his mom. I have always heard the Oedipus complex says that every man wants to kill his father and marry his mother. Ewe...

Emotionally Ben was married to his mom his whole life. I never mattered as much as she did. He wanted me to look like his mom and raise my kids like she would. Ultimately I think he felt she should take over mothering my kids because he knew he liked her more.

So I have mother in law issues. I really like my current mother in law though. She is a great person. But we all have our own baggage to deal with. The first cut is the deepest.

When I met Ben, the doors on his closet were all over his room. I asked, "What happened to your closet doors?" He said, "Oh my mom said it looks better that way." To me that proved she was crazy.

We lived with her for a few months before our first baby was born. She would pace the hallway at 2am and move things around. It may have been due to a medication she was on. I did not get why she wouldn't just go to sleep.

One time we were going on a road trip to CA so Ben could meet my parents. His mom texted and called him non stop to try to stop us from going. Maybe she feared that we would stay there forever. I wish we would have. Maybe our marriage would have lasted longer.

She babysat our two girls for one week so we could have a beach vacation. At the end of the week she texted me a text meant for her daughter. It said, "She didn't even ask how the girls were all week." I think she was gossiping trying to say I didn't care about my daughters at all. Gossip was her favorite hobby.

And here I am basically gossiping about her. The moral to this story is, don't be an annoying mother in law. Respect it that your child needs to move on. You should not run their life anymore. They need to bond with their mate and let go of you, so let them. Cut off those apron strings and let your kids be adults.

Not Working

 Every mom has to decide if it's better to stay home with her child or go work to make more money. I decided to not work. It seemed overall that my man didn't want me to, which is nice that he prefers that I relax at home. Partly I felt like he won't allow me to work, but oh well.

He mainly wants me to watch our baby as much as I can. Maybe he worried I would just forget about him and our baby and work all the time. I think a lot of women do that. I am glad I won't be doing that.

I woke up this morning super tired. It's hard when my baby wants to stay up late and then wake up early. He was up till 9pm and woke up at 7am. I guess that doesn't seem too crazy, but it's hard when he wakes up a lot in the middle of the night for a bottle. Then my stomach was hurting. I told Zach maybe that was a sign I'm not supposed to work for now. He said, "Yes it's a sign." So cute. :)

Anyways, I am glad overall I will not be working. I am glad I am doing what my man wants. I felt God tell me today, "If you care about submitting to your man, you won't even go to the interview." So I didn't.

We are doing ok on money. I wouldn't have had to work. I just wanted us to thrive instead of survive, but oh well. As long as we have what we need, that should be all that matters.

"Take the world, take it all but give me Jesus." -Red Rocks Worship

Skinny or Sick?

A big conflict in marriage is one person wanting the other to lose weight. It can be good to lose weight, but don't hurt yourself trying to do it.

"Scarlett Johansson has criticized the media for promoting an image that causes unhealthy diets and eating disorders among women." Good job to her.

3 people who got strangely skinny to the point of looking super sick were Justin Bieber, Michael Jackson and Celine Dion. Also Sandra Bullock looked overly thin in her last movie. I was somewhat proud of her for getting that thin but also it can be sad. Why does our culture think women have to be a size 2 to look cool or sexy? Why is it sexy to look like you hate food?

I suppose it looks sexy because the thought is you burn all the calories you eat by getting it on or cleaning your home. Men love a woman who likes sex and a clean home. That is why skinny bodies are appealing.

But then so many of us women feel like we can't eat so we can look hot like Hollywood actresses.

I wonder if I work again if I will gain or lose weight. I would hope to lose weight, but if I get free food I'll probably gain weight.

Ladies don't worry if you aren't a size 2. The good men don't care. At least they shouldn't care. It can be a spirit of death that leads women to starve themselves. Don't do that. Stay alive and healthy and looking well. Don't try to lose tons of weight too fast. It will only hurt you in the long run.

My Primi Baby

All my life I was worried I would have a primi baby someday. And it happened. My most recent baby was a pimi baby. He was born about a month early.

A couple family members came over when I was pregnant. They took my blood pressure and saw it was high. They rushed me to the hospital. Now I kind of resent them doing that. I wish I would have had a natural birth on time with my son, but you can't change the past.

When we got to a room, I told the nurses what I wanted to do. I was ready for an epidural and Pictocin to have my labor induced. I had been feeling I needed to get the baby out of me. I had terrible heartburn and arm pain. Both did get totally better after he came out.

I don't recommend every mom who has a painful pregnancy do that, but it was good overall for me. I have some regrets now. I think nursing would have worked out better if he was born at the proper timing.

The Pictocin didn't work so they did a C Section. He was skinny when he came out, but I got his weight up quickly.

If you ever have a baby, hopefully you can wait the full 9 months before having he or she come out. It isn't easy to be pregnant but at least you know it will be over at some point. It doesn't last forever.

Rejection

"I'm all out of love. I'm so lost without you." "You've lost that loving feeling oh...." "Do you really want to hurt me? Do you really want to make me cry?"

My mom rejected my crazy Sagittarius dad. I rejected my crazy Sagittarius ex-husband. I am a Sagittarius too, the less crazy kind. I worry sometimes that my bf will reject me too.

He works in a restaurant so I'm sure there are a lot of pretty women that he works with. I asked him about them a few times. He said they all have boyfriends, so that is great. That helps me sleep better at night.

But then I think back and wonder why he says no for intimacy half the time. Why didn't he spoon me when I asked? Is there a side woman?

There doesn't have to be a side woman. He could just be very non-romantic.

I wonder, why doesn't he show me that he loves me more?

He gets me lunch every day though. Every day when he wakes up, he asks me where I want lunch from. That is very sweet of him. He gives me cash each week to buy almost anything I want. Yet I still feel like he doesn't love me very much.

Sometimes I feel he does when he hugs me closer and squeezes me. I feel it when he wants to kiss me more than one time. I feel it when he looks at me with those loving eyes.

Most of the time though, I feel very little love coming from him. But maybe he feels very little love coming from me. Love is a reflection, it would seem. My attention is always on our baby now. I pour out on my love on our child. Maybe then I have less love left for my mate.

I suppose no one can express love in everything they do. Well I try to. Every time I clean our house I am telling him I love you. Every day I change his pillow case to say I love you. Every time I water our front yard I am telling him I love you. Sometimes I wash his truck.

It is important to show your lover how much you love them. If you don't often express it, that will make them very sad and lonely. Say I love you aloud and by doing things for them. That is how couples have always kept that spark going.

And don't ever make your mate feel rejected. Eventually they will stop desiring you as much if you constantly reject them.

Meg Ryan

Someone once told me I have a smile like Meg Ryan. I liked that compliment a lot. I think Meg Ryan was often conflicted with herself over who she wanted be married to.

I think the sweetest American actress has always been Meg Ryan. I think all us women wish we were more like her. There is a good interview of her with Oprah on YouTube. She divorced Dennis Quaid and was with Russel Crowe for a while. She said she didn't leave Dennis for Russel. She just wanted to leave her marriage. She said it wasn't a good marriage. They had a son together. I can only imagine what Dennis was like as a dad. If you have seen the movie "Yours, Mine and Ours" it makes you wonder if he was like that. A general commanding his family around. Oh dear....

I was just thinking how she was in 3 movies with Tom Hanks. I think both of them are Christian. You can see it in their eyes. It is really too bad they didn't ever get married. They were in Sleepless in Seattle first, which I am going to watch again today. I loved them so much in You've Got Mail. I have seen that movie many times. I love that it's about bookstores since I was an English major. They are the cutest couple in any movie in that one. And they were in Joe Vs. The Volcano together. Most people don't know about that movie. It is a bit odd. Joe hates his job and quits. A rich guy gives him money to go to an island. He is almost a sacrifice for the natives there to their god but he makes it out alive. It is about living a life you love and not just doing the same old routine that you hate every day. It was a great movie.

I read Meg Ryan's wikipedia the other day and I found it interesting that after her divorce, all of her movies didn't do very well in the box office. Why was that? Either the movie scripts she picked were not that good, or the public was mad at her for divorcing Dennis and boycotted her movies. How sad. One movie only made 150K. That is almost nothing for a movie. It was called Serious Moonlight. I saw that and I liked it. I think it's worth watching. It is free on YouTube. It's about a woman who discovers her man is going to leave her for a younger woman. She refuses to let him go and tapes him to a chair until he changes his mind. He agrees to give her a baby. A year later he realizes the whole thing was a set up to make him fall in love with her again. He felt dooped. He probably wished he had run off with the younger woman.

Everyone wants a younger person. I suppose because it makes you feel younger to be with someone younger. My current man is younger than me. I am happy I finally got a young guy. :) My ex was 4 years older but when we separated, he looked about 20 years older than me. 😵 His hair was all grey and he had a lot of wrinkles already. I suppose that was from smoking for 25 years. It definitely ages someone a lot faster. Also he stressed out over everything. That also aged him a ton faster.

Meg Ryan it seems did the same thing. She was married to Dennis who was 8 years older than her. I can imagine he was bossy with her. The older person is almost always bossy with the younger person. I try to not be bossy with my man, but I'm sure I come off as bossy very often.

When she left Dennis, she went for Russel Crowe who was 2 years younger than her. I bet he was a lot more fun than her old, mean, grumpy husband. I used to call my ex grumpy bear often, because he was usually very grumpy. Now I am the grumpy older person, sometimes. I suppose it is just how things go. The older you get, the more grumpy you become. Oh well.

I have a few Meg Ryan movies I haven't seen yet. I hope they are worth seeing. And I hope she gets to do a few more really great movies before her career is officially over. Go Meg Ryan! You are great!

Desire Less

The message often in movies is what you have isn't good enough. Go try to find a better mate. In the movie The Stepford Wives there is a TV show titled "I Can Do Better."

Or maybe what you have is as good as it gets. Maybe you already have all that you need and want. Just learn to be happy where you are. It might seem like the grass could be greener on the other side, but what if it's not.

Learn to love what you already have. You loved it once. You can still love it now, if you desire to.

People do not fall out of love. They fall out of forgiveness. Understanding. Loving the other person despite the things you don't like about them. Loving without harsh criticism. You may have to come to realize they aren't perfect, but neither are you. Maybe things they do bother you. You most likely bother them too, in many ways. They overlook those things in you. Why can't you overlook those things in them? That is what they deserve.

Learn to love judgement free again. Let go of the bitterness and skepticism and jaded mentality. Things can always be great if you decide to keep them great.

PMS

I have really bad PMS. I think what happens is I get a surge of testosterone. I feel on my PMS days how men feel every day, it would seem. I understand why they drink. They need that to stay calm.

For me it helps to get more exercise to get all that energy out. I used to play basketball a lot. Now I go for walks.

If you know women who get bad PMS, suggest that they take a walk when they feel irritable. And limit caffeine intake on those days. That will help.

Us women tend to act in a rash way when PMS'ing. I yelled at my ex about going to the ER 5 years ago. He had pain that he imagined was cancer. I felt he was just being paranoid. That day of me flipping out over that ended our marriage. It was falling apart already, because he kept thinking I was cheating even though I never did, but that really killed any love that was left. It was this testosterone overdose from PMS that caused that.

This is most likely why tons of divorces happen. The woman might act possessed due to PMS. But it's not demons, it's hormones.

Maybe someday soon I'll get a hysterectomy so I won't have hormone fluctuations anymore.

Young Love

The first two things that taught me about love were the movie The Little Mermaid and the song The Power of Love.

I wanted to find a guy to love like Ariel loved Prince Eric. I wanted to cuddle someone like Celine Dion sang about.

Then I grew up and realized most adult love is a bit different than those two images in my head. Most adult couples are more like friends who sometimes are attracted to each other. The spark doesn't stay alive for very long.

You have to be a responsible adult. That means you realize you can't get whatever you want. Cuddling rarely works due to snoring. Your prince does not stay totally perfect forever.

What did you anticipate love would be like as a child? How different is love for you now?

I hope you figure out ways to keep that flame burning. Don't let the fire go out, because it is sad when it does.

Growing Up

Almost every Disney movie is about a girl coming of age, leaving home, setting out on her own. I suppose they were giving us young girls a warning. "Someday you will have to leave the comfort of your home and start your own home. This is just a fact of life." There are girls and women who stay at home forever, but if we all did that, the human species would cease to exist. In order for humans to keep breeding, Disney wanted to help get girls ready for growing up. The message to us girls was basically, "Go find your man and fall in love. Keep the economy going."

In the Little Mermaid she couldn't wait to be part of his world. In Tangled she couldn't wait to get out of that tower. In Moana she couldn't wait to get out on the main ocean. In Anastasia she couldn't wait to get to Paris. In Aladdin she couldn't wait to escape the palace. In Beauty and the Beast she wanted more than her provincial life, whatever that meant.

Most girls grow up comfortable and protected. Then one day we venture out on our own and see the world!

When I was in my teens, I couldn't wait to leave home and go to college. Disney prepared me very well for that. I couldn't wait to meet my prince charming. I had a few princes. I don't know if I would say any of them were charming. I suppose they tried. My current man is the most charming guy so far. Good job to him. :)

When I was young, I couldn't wait to see the world, and I did. The parts I really wanted to see. I got to live in Hawaii and Australia and visit Alaska and the Bahamas and Taiwan and India. I almost went to England. I had my share of adventures for sure. I still hope to have some. Part of me just wants to stay in my house forever and never do anything adventurous ever again. My mom just got Covid on her Hawaii cruise so that might be why. It is better to stay in one place perhaps. Just be safe.

What adventures have you always wanted to go on? Maybe you should. And I hope you don't ever get Covid.

Satan Destroys Families

 "Be sober-minded; be watchful. Your adversary the devil prowls around like a roaring lion, seeking someone to devour."

Most people totally ignore Satan, which is naive. When their life falls apart, they have no idea why. They let Satan take control of their mind in some way. They gave him a foothold. They talked with demons without realizing that was what they were doing.

If any thought feels like a mean or discouraging thought, that is Satan. Tell him to stop talking to you.

 Maybe you like having an entity to talk to. Talk to the Holy Spirit instead. How do you know the difference? If you love others and you constantly want to listen to sermons or worship music, you are most likely talking with the Holy Spirit. If you hate yourself and others, you are probably talking with demons.

Keep your mind clean of Satan and demons. You will greatly regret it later if you don't.

Don't Pray to Die

So 5 months ago I prayed to die. I was pregnant and hated being pregnant. My heartburn was terrible. My arms felt like they were on fire due to tendonitis.

I was trying to get rich, or save the world, writing a new book every week. Mainly I just wanted to help people get better.

So eventually I got worn out. And I wanted God to kill me. 🙁 So he gave me pre-clampsia. That was him basically slowly killing me while hoping I would change my mind. My vision got really bad. I thought I was going blind. My blood pressure got crazy high.

Blindness actually is a biblical punishment. Saul went blind before he got saved. Then he was healed. God was essentially punishing me for praying to die. Well also he took my prayer seriously.

I would think that is a common occurrence. How many people actually want to stay alive for 50 more years? And if you do, why? For any of us who believe in heaven, why would we want to stay here any longer?

Because God prefers that we do. That is why we have to. I don't know why he makes us all stay alive. Well I do know why, so we can save the lost. It seems like an impossible task at times. That is why most don't even bother to save or help anyone. We don't have many warriors left in the world. ☐ Most people are lazy and scared all the time. So they never try to save the world.

Go save the world! You can do it.

But try to not get overwhelmed with your effort. You can help a few people. Maybe not everyone will get helped, but a special few can be saved. So try, please. I don't want to be the only one trying to save the world.

Peace

"As far as it depends on you, live at peace with all people."

There is no need to start drama. Just be silent if you are upset. Take a nap. Eat a good meal. Think for awhile before you say anything. Take a walk. Watch a good movie. Not every thought you have needs to be said. God reveals things to us at times to show us what to pray for, but we do not have to discuss every little thing we are upset about.

It is better to stay at peace with others than to start drama.

A good book about this is Speaking the Truth in Love. It says how we need to be assertive, but not passive or aggressive. If you clearly state how you feel or what you want, that can save you from a lot of fighting. If you never express what you want, you are being passive. Eventually the resentment will build up and you will just leave the relationship. If you lash out every time you are upset, that is being aggressive. You will probably scare the other person away eventually. You have to find the middle ground and keep the peace. Say how you feel but in a calm way.

Say what you need to say but don't be a maneater, or a woman eater. That is in reference to the 80's song that you all should listen to.

Be a Giver

"Whatever you do to the least of these, you have done to me," Jesus said.

What do you do for those that no one else seems to care about? Did you know any way you serve them is like serving Jesus?

If you are kind to your animals or homeless animals, it is like you are serving Jesus himself.

Whoever the least of these is to you, serve them. Be kind to them. Be patient with them.

"Those who deserve love the least need it the most." Who do you know who probably doesn't deserve love at all? Give them the most love of anyone, because who knows what mark you will make on the world if you do that.

Jesus said don't only love those who love you. Love those who can't or will not love you back. Then great will be your reward in heaven.

Sagittarius

My sign is the Sagittarius. Other people who are my sign tend to be a bit crazy. This has always made me a bit sad to be the sign that I am. On the upside though, Brad Pitt is a Sagittarius.

Crazy Sagittarius people....

My ex was one and he went insane.

My dad was one and he was a repeat sex predator.

My step brother was one and he had a strange desire to nail virgins. Very mean.

My grandpa was one and he physically abused my uncle and insulted me about my weight a few times.

My co-worker had an ex who was one. She told him she was praying to die and that some other woman might help him take care of their kids.

I know a lady who is one who is in a psychosis state and is on way too many medications.

I have heard of another Sagittarius who had very erratic crazy behavior.

And then here I am. I try to be normal. I guess the crazy thing I did was travel a lot.

I think for us Sagittarius people, if we don't get to travel a lot, we go crazy. Cabin fever perhaps? We love to explore new places.

It is the strongest sign in many ways. It is referred to as the warrior sign. I have always felt like a warrior, but I try to be compliant when I can and subdued.

If you know a Sagittarius, be patient with us. We can't help being a little wild. We were born to be wild, but we can be a good wild.

Number 8 Grandchild

 My mom is visiting today to meet my baby boy. I need to remember to take pictures of the two of them.

This baby is her 8th grandchild. Her first one was born 22 years ago when my brother had his son. My step brothers each had 2 kids. Then this is my 3rd child. I win! Lol Because I had 3 kids. Most people stop after 2, which is good to do. I had a third because my first 2 were withheld from me. Locked in a dungeon by their evil grandmother. Someday maybe they will be free. May they feel free at some point soon in Jesus name amen.

Life is crazy. You never know what could happen. Hopefully my family will have some stability now. Thank you God for giving us a second chance. May things be happy and greater this time with my new family. May we all love each other the way you love us God. May

we stay calm and humble and kind. Thank you God for family. May
we be a strong family in the future.

Break Ups

I have broken up with guys that I was with many, many times. I was
with a guy off and on in high school. I kept breaking up with him
because he didn't act like a Christian. He was raised in church, but I
saw him as a bad boy because he smoked and drank and had multiple
girlfriends. I think almost all guys are bad boys, but I didn't realize
that then.

A guy I dated in college I was very in love with, but I broke up with
him to focus on school more. I wish I would have just dropped out of
college and married him. He was a great guy.

The next guy I broke up with, because I told him "I love you" and he
said he didn't love me. What an idiot.

The next guy broke up with me, because I didn't like shopping. It was
also because he was Pentecostal, and I was Baptist. That was the
cause of the break-up in my previous marriage too. I saw that coming
from the beginning, because of this former break up. I thought we
might work out, but Baptists should never try being with
Pentecostals. They are way too different, in how they see God and in
their way of living life. I always felt like I believed in a totally different
God than my ex did. His God was a get rich quick and never stay sick
God. My God was a God that forces you to grow through staying sick
and being poor at times, a God that wants to keep you humble. A lot
of people believe in a God of their own imagination. You can't really
be saved unless you believe in the God of the Bible.

With my next bf, I broke up with him because he was very mean to his
3 year old son. I didn't get why he lost his patience so much. It was

very sad to be around and to watch. So I moved on. Also he told me he was gay in the past. He had a bf for a few months. That grossed me out, so I could not fully love him after knowing about that.

My next bf I may have stayed with forever, but he went to jail. He missed a few doses of his medication and decided to shoot up a building of his former employer. Our savings was running out and he didn't get paid by this former employer. He wanted to "teach him a lesson," so he shot 6 windows in his business. He went to jail for about 7 months.

My next bf was Jewish. I should have known it wouldn't last, because Jewish people usually only hook up with other Jewish people. It mainly was his horrible temper that kept me breaking up with him. I must have broken up with him 5 times or more. We kept getting back together because there was love there, but it was an odd love. We were more like siblings than lovers. I still pray for him when I think of him. I hope he will have a happy life someday.

Then I was single for 6 months and had my own apartment. That was the most peaceful time of my life. I very much enjoyed having my own place. But I got lonely, so I decided to find yet another bf.

I met my current man via online dating. I was ready to start family number 2, so we did. I don't think I will ever have a reason to break up with him. He is Christian, very sweet, has a nice body, and he is a hard worker. I love him very much! And he is younger than me yay.... I have always wanted a younger guy and I got one. Good job to me.

Hopefully there will be no more break ups and I will be happy to live with my current man forever.

May God help you all to stay with your person and to be happy with them forever. You can do it. I believe in you.

Sneaking Around

Every person who is with a mate sneaks around on them in some way. Some women hide packages they order from their mate. A ton of men watch porn at least once a day, and their woman has no clue.

With an ex I had, I would pretend to be working late but just go sit in my car at the park. I didn't want to go home yet. I hated going home to him and his son. He yelled at his son a lot. It was the saddest and most stressful living set up I had ever had.

My first bf and I never snuck around in any way. We gave each other freedom to do anything we wanted to do. It's not really love if you don't let each other have total freedom. Trust your mate. They are most likely smart enough to do the right thing.

A lot of men and women sneak smoking, or drinking, or other drugs. I still think one of my exes was sneaking doing drugs the whole 7 years I was with him. He certainly acted like he did.

Probably in half of relationships there is a man or a woman on the side. Every time I had a job, there was always some guy I liked at work, even if I had my own man at the time. This is why women should just stay home and raise the kids. But then us women are always worried that our man has a woman on the side at work. My only words of comfort on that are, "If it's meant to be it'll be. Baby just let it be."

In the movie The Waitress she sneaks in hiding money all over the house so she can escape from her verbally abusive husband. I used to say all people are just with someone until someone better comes along. That is a true statement in most relationships.

As long as you treat your mate with respect, you won't have to worry about them wanting to be with someone else. Affairs happen when a person feels sad, threatened, alone or forgotten within a relationship. They stopped being happy at some point, with their mate and just in general. They think some new life set up will make them happy. Will it? It may or it may not. No life situation is perfect. We all just have to take what God gives us. No one is perfectly happy. My advice to you is stop hoping you can be perfectly happy. In heaven you will be, but never on this earth. It is never going to happen. Sorry if that pops your bubble.

The more you feverishly chase happiness, the more it eludes you. Give up the chase. If you are 70% happy now, that should be good enough.

Decide to love what you have and forget about everything else. And try to never sneak around on your mate. It will only stress you out, and what you are doing probably isn't worth it.

Fruits and Veggies

 I realized today the gospel writers never record Jesus eating fruits or veggies. He only seemed to eat fish and bread, and he drank wine. That would be like us eating only pizza and drinking juice or smoothies, which I did for about 3 years while working at Papa John's.

Every guy I have been with has zero interest in fruits or veggies. That always frustrates me. I want to say to them, "Don't you care about not dying early?" They could say back, "Awe you want me to be your work mule forever?" ☺ Maybe most men want to die early. Ladies, let's give our men a reason to want to stay alive for a long time. Try to be more nice to the men you are around.

Women are better at thinking of the future. Men for some reason don't realize that what they do now affects their future a lot.

Eat fruit and veggies. Maybe Jesus didn't eat a ton of healthy food but he was God. His health was perfect no matter what. We all need to eat more healthy to stay alive for a long time, and to feel better as long as we are alive.

Divorce and Demons

 I just realized that my mom most likely divorced my dad for the same reason that I divorced my ex. Both my dad and my ex became possessed. Not possessed like in the movies. But they both had several demons messing with them that they couldn't shake off. My ex had demons talking to him all day, every day about me, trying to turn him against me. My dad had demons telling him he would never amount to anything so he should just give up. He stopped wanting to attend church or go to counseling. He started drinking two beers before bed instead of one. He was kind of flirty with the women at church. They were all behaviors that were self-sabotaging. It seemed like he wanted my mom to give up on him, and she did.

I said to my ex at one point, "I give up." It was too much for me to try to prove my innocence to him while demons kept telling him that I did bad things. He kept thinking I was cheating, but I never did. He thought I said terrible things that I never said. One thing was he said that I said his ex slept with all his co-workers. He must have asked me 10 times why I said that. I said, "I never said that," but he refused to believe me. I don't know if he heard that in bad dreams that he had or he was tripping out while he was awake. A few people I talked to said it sounded like he was doing meth. I have no idea ultimately. He may have been taking drugs, or it was just the demons that caused all of his delusions. People on drugs often attract demons through the drugs, in that they let their guard down so demons can mess with them easier. That may be why it seemed like he was on something. But sadly for him, he didn't need to be on something to let the demons in to pester him.

We all need to be careful of that. Don't let demons mess up your life like they did with my ex. In a way maybe his life is peachy keen now because he is not the sole bread winner for his daughters or me. His mom is helping him a lot, but I'm sure she resents it. And he will probably never get to have sex again. Once demons take over a person's mind, it is very difficult to get the demons to leave. I remember Joyce Meyer saying she did a deliverance ministry for a while. She would cast demons out of people, but before they even got back to their chair, the demons were right back in them.

In order for anyone to get free of demons, they have to want the demons to leave. Why do so many people not want their demons to leave? They are lonely and bored. That seems silly to us normal people. Why can't they find ways to entertain themselves other than talking to demons all day? I have no idea. They want someone to keep them company. It should be God, or a good friend, but they refuse to connect with either God or good people. That is very sad, obviously. But the demons are why they don't have any friends, because it is obvious something is wrong with them. But then that rejection from people makes them more attached to their demons. They think if they let the demons go, they will have no one, but they are deceived.

It is hard to know what to do with such people. It is good to try to help them, but we all know the saying, "Don't try to save a drowning person or you too might drown." That is why I finally gave up on my ex. I felt bad about it of course, but everyone has their limit of what they can handle. You can only give away so much.

If you are around any possessed people, or people that seem disturbed, just leave them to themselves. Don't let them bring you down. Don't let them make you get possessed too. It can happen. Don't let them ruin your life like they have ruined their own. Keep yourself safe. For some people it is almost impossible to save them. Stay in the light and stay away from the darkness and dark people. That is the wisest thing to do.

Good luck to you all. May God give you discernment as you try to decide who should be in your life and who should not be.

Perspective

 Your perspective on any situation is key. You can wake up thinking your day will be great. You will then make it great. You can feel dread over what you have to do that day, but what is the point to that?

Feelings can be good. If you really don't want to do something, don't do it. Changing your perspective might help though. Think that it will go well, whatever it is, and it most likely will.

Maybe you have a date. Picture it going well. Maybe you have a job interview. Picture yourself getting hired right away.

Your mind will create your future. What you see yourself doing is what you probably will do. Our imagination dictates our thoughts and those dictate our actions and those dictate our future. If you want your future to be peaceful, think peaceful thoughts. Think happy thoughts. Don't let negative thoughts ruminate in your mind too long.

You have to switch your attitude if you feel negative. Playing fun music can help. Watching something inspiring on YouTube can help. Try to keep your thoughts positive if you want your life to be positive.

For example, I need to get a new battery for my car today. It has not been starting very well. Granted the car is 20 years old and the heat this summer has been crazy. Maybe it killed my battery just from it being so hot outside. Old cars just need greater care. I will imagine that it will go well. The line won't be long. They will have the battery I need, and it won't be overpriced. And they will think my car looks cute even though I stupidly covered it in contact paper 2 years ago. I did that to re-create my other car I had like this one. My first car was a white Toyota Echo. I bought this car 3 years ago. It looked the same except the outside was grey. I decided to make it white, but the contact paper looks kind of silly. Oh well. It can't be undone.

Today I might go buy more flowers. I will picture myself getting the most gorgeous flowers for my outside area ever. I will believe that they will not die in this summer heat, but they will have a long life.

If you stay home or if you work, have a positive perspective about it. If you work, you get to be social all day and that is great. If you stay home, you get to not be bothered by many people and that is great too.

Whatever your lot in life is, be grateful for it. There is always something about it you can appreciate.

Forgive Them

I think a lot of marriage conflict is due to anger that each has at the opposite sex. I used to make bracelets a lot. I am sure that is the main reason I have arthritis issues and that triggered the pre-clampsia that I had. I put on a bracelet one time, "Forgive Him." I felt like that was a word from the Lord. I have so many him's that I need to forgive. Almost every him I have known, I need to forgive.

My dad molested me. My brother did too. Another older guy did. All the guys who broke my heart I need to forgive. I still need to forgive my ex for letting his mind go insane and causing our family break up. My grandpa for speaking harshly at times. Guys that I worked with who were demeaning toward me.

I am sure every guy has a lot of hers that he needs to forgive. The start of most relationships is both people talking about their exes and how they were hurt by them. You help each other heal from all the previous pain. You assure each other that you will never hurt them like that other person did.

There is always so much pain to heal from.

May God help you all heal from your own pain from the opposite sex. Let those people go. Don't let them continue to hurt you by remembering what they did to you. Forgive and forget, when you are ready to.

Kids Cause a Goodbye

 Before I got pregnant I felt like God said to me, "He doesn't realize this will make him have to say goodbye to you." That was in reference to me getting pregnant and having Zach's baby. Why did God say that? Not that I would leave physically, but we barely see each other now.

Before I had our baby I would water the yard in the mornings, take a bath, and then come and cuddle with him. We pretty much never cuddle anymore. I always only cuddled with him in the mornings because he didn't snore then, for whatever reason. At night my man snores as loud as an airplane.

Now he has to work tons. He works 14 hour days 3 days a week, 7 hour days 3 days a week and only gets one day off. On that one day he is so tired all he wants to do is drink and sleep all day.

So children have a way of making couples say goodbye to each other, even though they are still technically together. This is why a lot of couples wait to have kids or never have kids. They know they will barely see each other afterwards. But that is life.

When I was younger I never wanted to have kids actually. One of my exes convinced me by saying, "Well who will take care of you when you are old?" I was like, "Ok, that is a good reason to have kids."

To all you fellow parents, I know how you feel if you miss your mate. Someday you will get to hang out with them again, when the kids are grown. Or when they are teens, and they want to have their own life apart from you. Hang in there and stay strong.

My Testimony

I was raised in a very religious family. I say religious because my mom was Christian but my dad was just religious. They were involved in a church called "the Local Church" for a long time, which was very legalistic. The people may have looked good on the outside and said all the right stuff, but it was mostly goodness out of competition or fear I think.

My dad molested me for awhile in my childhood. I could never wrap my mind around how he could be Christian and do that, but he wasn't Christian, he was just religious. I have had a lot of anger at my mom throughout my lifetime about all that, mainly just at the fact that she married my dad. I felt she should have taken more time to really judge his character before marrying him, since obviously he turned out to be a bit crazy. He was analyzed by psychiatrists who said he was "highly intelligent but with a skewed sense of reality." That skewed sense was that he thought it was his job to teach me everything about life, including sexuality. Very skewed indeed.

He went to jail when I was 6 because I told my mom about something he did. She did not know the whole time what was happening. He was only in jail for a short time and our family reunited after he got out, which I also had anger at my mom about as an adult. If it were me, I would have never spoken to him again.

But then when I was 9 my parents divorced, praise God. Although that divorce was a bit hard on me. I started getting into a lot of trouble, shoplifting and drinking and smoking from about 12 to 14. Mainly it was because I felt that I was bad due to what happened to me so I thought I might as well act bad.

When I was 14 my mom and I moved to California from Nebraska to be by her parents. Praise God for that because from then on my grandma was a very strong and very positive influence in my life. She helped me see that I needed to do better and that God had a great plan for my life, despite what happened to me. I felt like she really believed in me, that I could do anything and be anything. So I did. I went on a mission's trip at 14 to India. I joined all the leadership teams at my church. I was in tons of AP classes in high school and a debate club and choir and basketball. I did everything I could do. I love a quote I heard once, "The most reprobate sinners become the most devout saints." I think it's because the energy you put into being bad you then put into doing good and helping others.

Then I went to Biola for college, a private Christian school. I kind of had the wind taken out of my sails there. I think I felt less than the other kids who all seemed to come from perfect families. I felt kind of like the black sheep there all four years. I also had lots of anxiety about what people thought of me and my grades. But I did learn a ton about the Bible and God there and I praise God for that.

After college I mostly worked at jobs helping kids. I felt like my calling in life was to help other kids have a really happy childhood since I didn't. I have heard "Your greatest ministry comes from your greatest pain." My greatest pain was that most of my young life was not happy at all, so I wanted to create happiness for as many kids as I could. I ran games at summer camps, tried teaching and did lots of tutoring. I tried to encourage as many kids as I could, like my grandma always had encouraged me.

At 25 I met a wonderful Christian guy. We got engaged, but when I was 27 he died due to drinking while on to many prescriptions. That started a war inside me kind of against prescription drugs and doctors. That time of grieving over his death was a very, very hard time for me. I never questioned my faith though. I only pressed harder into God in that time and started writing in my new blog a ton. His death made me realize even more how little time we all have, and that I could die any day. I felt all the more that I needed to start doing as much as I could to help others and change the world, as much as I could.

When I was 28 I met my ex-husband online. We had two little girls who were total angels. We divorced 3 years ago due to his mental health problems. He may have just been scientifically Schitzophrenic, or demons were pestering him in his mind. Whatever it was, we could not stay together. I did not feel safe living with him anymore, due to his involvement in Charismania. I felt that type of church was full of witchcraft and as a result, he seemed to become possessed.

About 9 years ago I started making something I call "Jesus Packets" that have bracelets, candy and a Bible tract. I think my motivation for those is that if I can't save my dad, maybe I can help to save many others. I think I have made about 8,000 of those so far. Hopefully those are making a difference. My goal in life has always been to push away the darkness as much as I can and shine as much light in this world as I can in any way I can, through music or making craft things or my blog writing. Hopefully God has taken every effort I have made and multiplied it's effects like Jesus did with the bread and the fish.

About 10 months ago I met my current sweetie. We will start a family soon. I am very excited. We both went to Christian school for awhile growing up. We feel like a good match and God willing, we will stay together forever.

If you have never prayed to receive the free gift of Jesus' salvation, say this prayer, "God thank you for sending Jesus to die for me. Holy Spirit please come into my heart and transform me into the person God wants me to be."

Here is a good tip for you all. Something great to do in your free time is to start a Bible study habit. Search any topic on the website OpenBible.com. You can read every Bible verse that exists on any topic you may want to learn more about. May God bless you and your family!

About the Author:

Lisa Bedrick was born and raised in Orange County, CA. She currently lives in West Texas. She was saved at age 14 and went to a private Christian college. She has a B.A. in English. God is number one in her life. She met her man, Zach through online dating. He is a great Christian guy. Soon they will start a family.